MIND FOR PEACE

Mindful living for today

Balboa Press books may be ordered through booksellers or by contacting:

Balboa Press
A Division of Hay House
1663 Liberty Drive
Bloomington, IN 47403
www.balboapress.com
1 (877) 407-4847

ISBN: 978-1-9822-1783-9 (sc)
ISBN: 978-1-9822-1782-2 (hc)
ISBN: 978-1-9822-1784-6 (e)

Library of Congress Control Number: 2018914395

Print information available on the last page.

Balboa Press rev. date: 01/18/2019

BALBOA.
PRESS
A DIVISION OF HAY HOUSE

For my and our children

Dear Reader,

This book was motivated by my desire to share with you the beauty of our world. It is about our *awareness*, not only in the living but also in the being, that together with our ability to love nurtures our path in life. It is my hope that it will inspire you to live your life through the widest lens and from upon the highest tree top.

My hope is that with every page you will feel the joy that surrounds you—for each detail of life is a blessing.

Thank you.

Tulia Maria de Sousa

Awareness of our surrounding world is about *being mindful* of each moment as it happens. This awareness allows us to increase our focus, manage our emotions, make better decisions, and empathize more profoundly in our relationships.

It reflects a clarity of mind that enables us to connect with our senses and truly see the blue tranquil sky above us or hear the warm caring voice of a friend.

How do we learn to become more aware?

We begin by learning about our breath. When we think of our needs, we may think: eating, drinking, praying or maybe even working or playing—yet we often forget about our breath. Our breath is a miracle of the human body. When we are aware of our breath we are reminded of the privilege of being alive in a world where true beauty can be found. This thought provides us with a welcoming sense of calmness.

Our breath is also our anchor in moments of anxiety and stress.

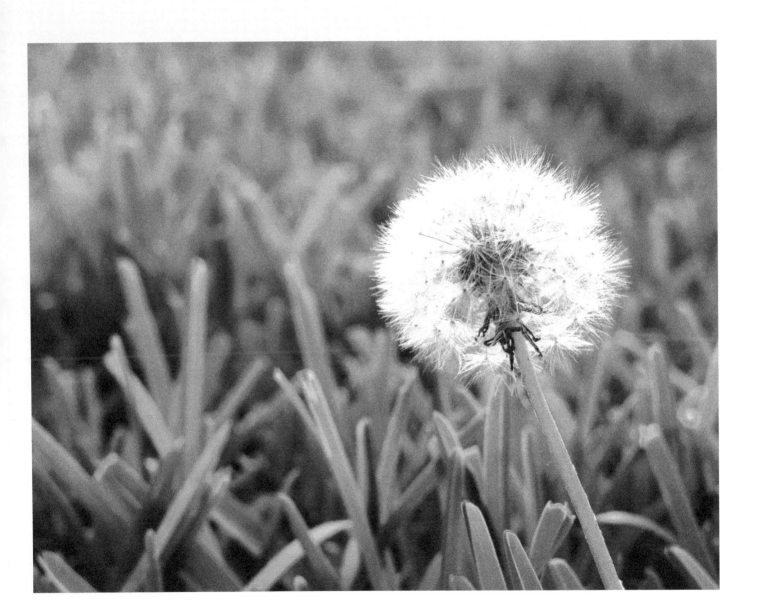

However, just as important is our awareness of our inner self, subconscious or soul. Real beauty lays from within ourselves as our outer beauty is in constant transformation with the passing of time.

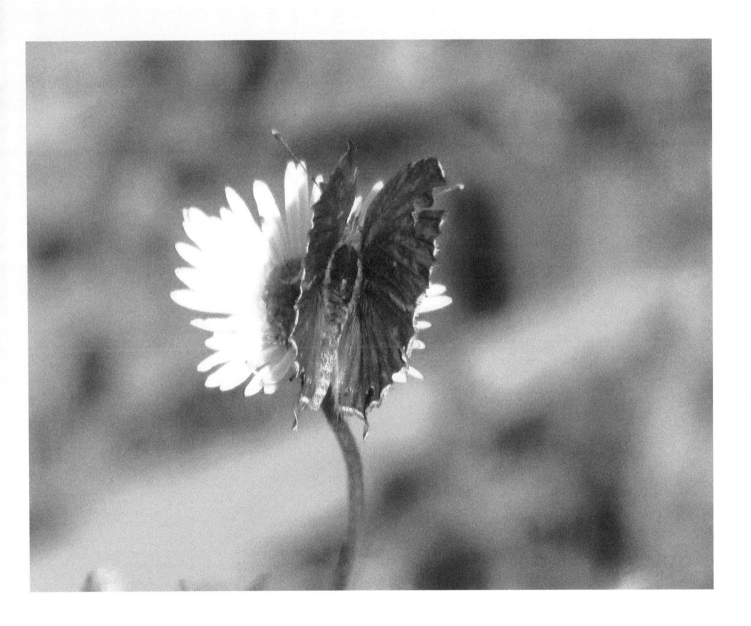

How do we reconcile our notion of beauty with notions of beauty that are given to us by society? By being mindful of our thoughts and complete awareness of ourselves.

Sounds difficult? We need to want to and believe we can—for if we are able to see the soul, true beauty is found.

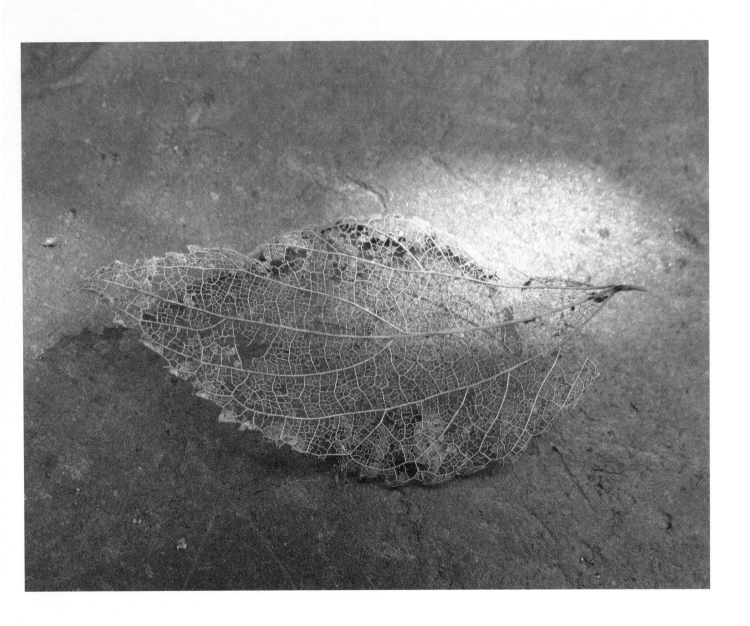

With our awareness, we come to understand that love is the greatest gift of all.

Can you imagine a world where there is no love?

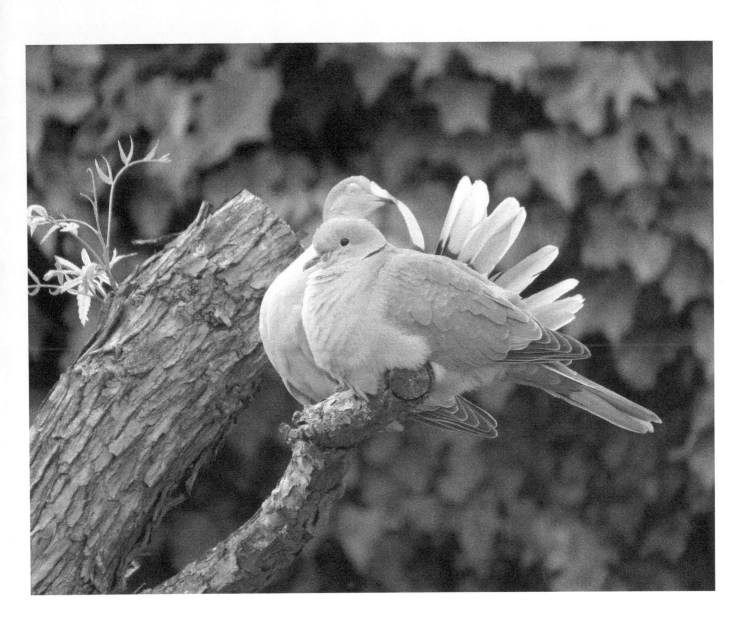

With love comes our faith and our ability to work and live together. Both within our differences and on our common ground—our world: earth, moon, stars and universe.

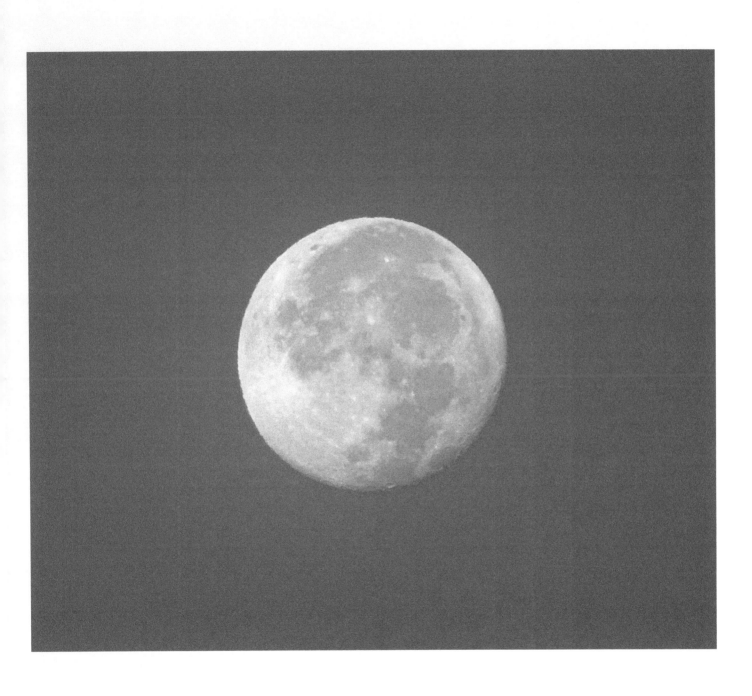

The art of mindfulness, or of being aware, is a life long path. From the moment we are born our lives are a constant journey—the ripples of the water gentle and rough as we glide through the seas.

Ultimately, this is our challenge: to sail in peace. Mindfulness is a sail.

Mindful living implies love, kindness and gratitude.

We are grateful for the sun that shines warmly on our backs, our family and friends that make us laugh, the food that nourishes our bodies, and the farmers that grow our crops.

It is upon this foundation that our resilience will grow and flourish.

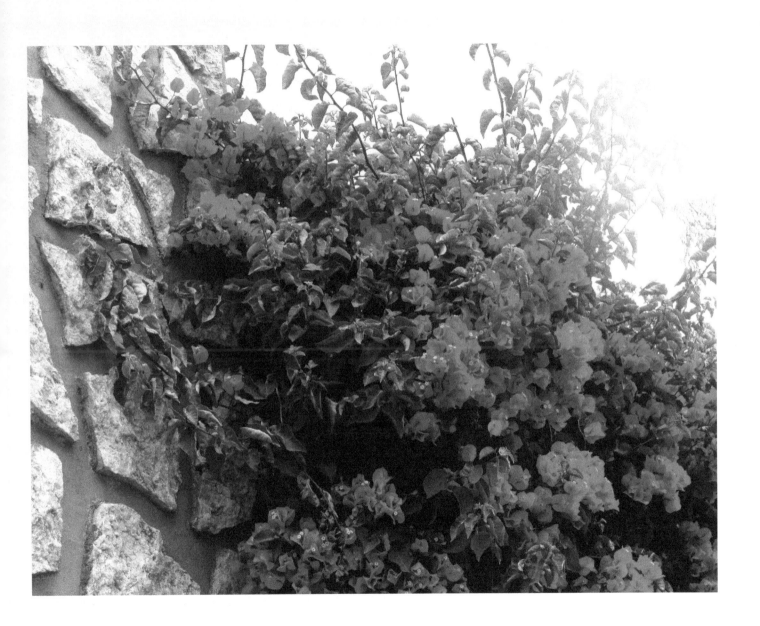

Our pets add real essential beauty to our lives. There is so much we can learn from them for their ability to love unconditionally is inspiring.

Let us care for the animals that share our planet with us.

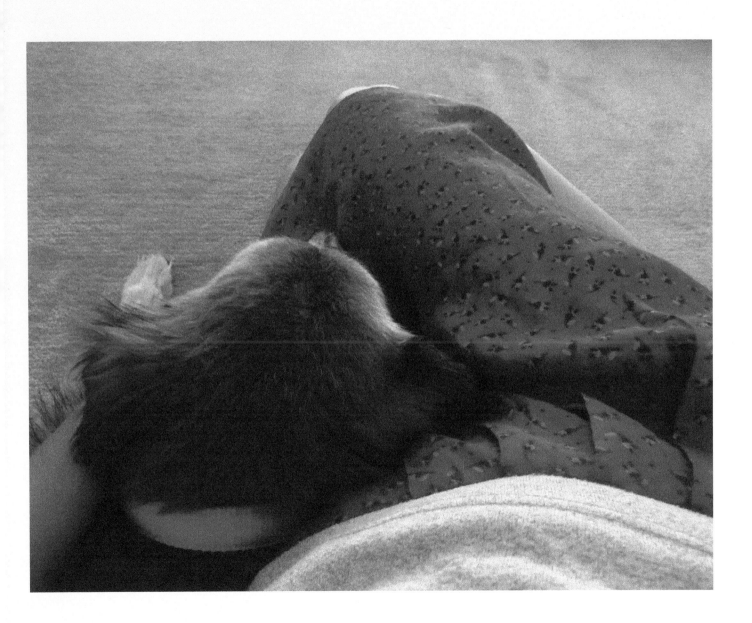

A child to a parent, a student to a teacher, a grandchild to a grandparent, a friend to a friend. Mindful learning of respect and love shines light upon our paths. It helps us live within our communities in harmony with ourselves and each other.

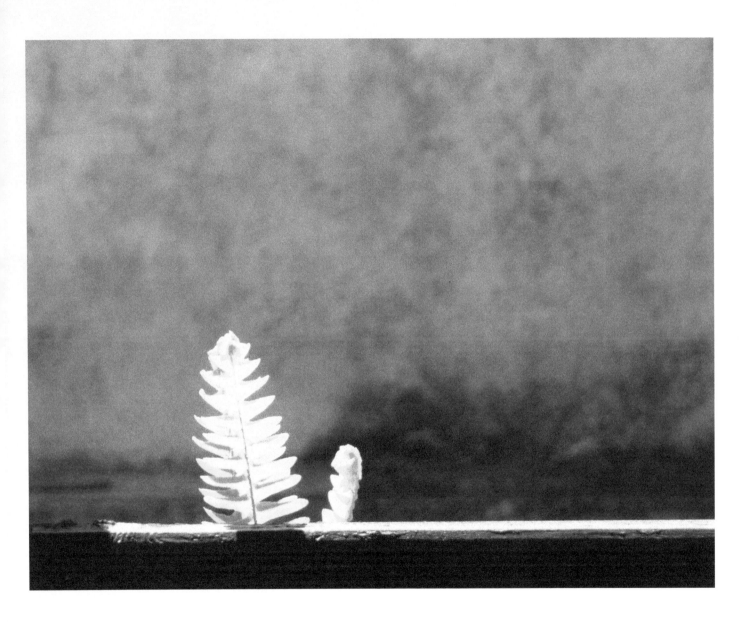

Unfortunately, bullying can be a problem among the young and old, where those who seem smaller or insignificant are subject to intolerance and unkindness. Let us journey upon our earth mindfully with love and awareness, and remember that all that lays before us is special.

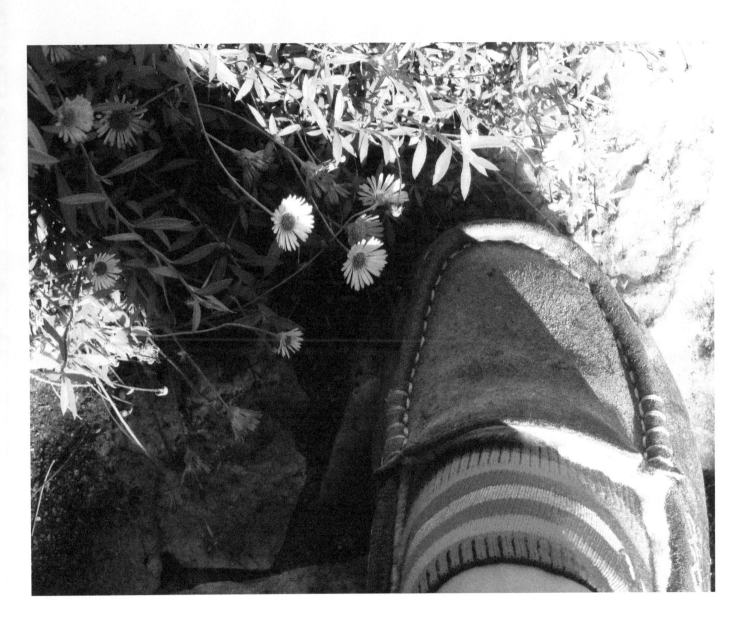

Our shoe size, type or color is no measure of wisdom. It is the gentle firmness upon which we mindfully stand on solid ground that is the measure.

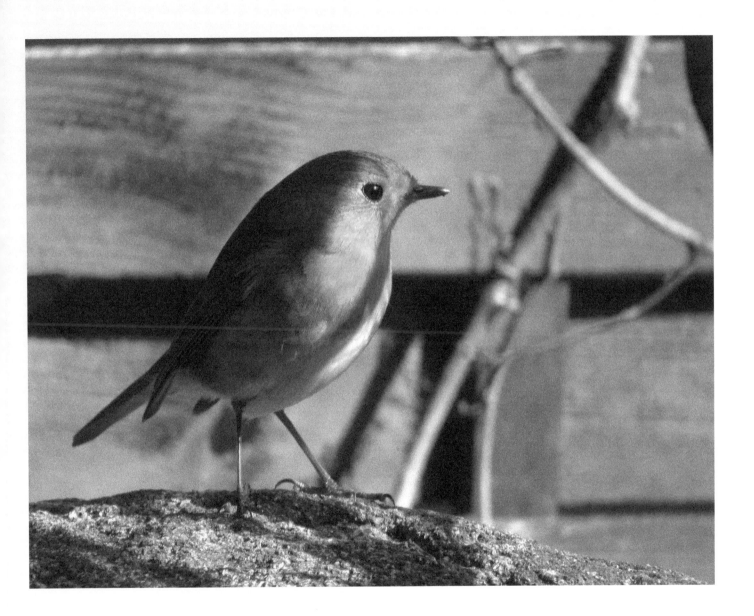

As light shines peacefully on our paths we will be able to truly see, hear, smell, feel and touch the wonders of our world.

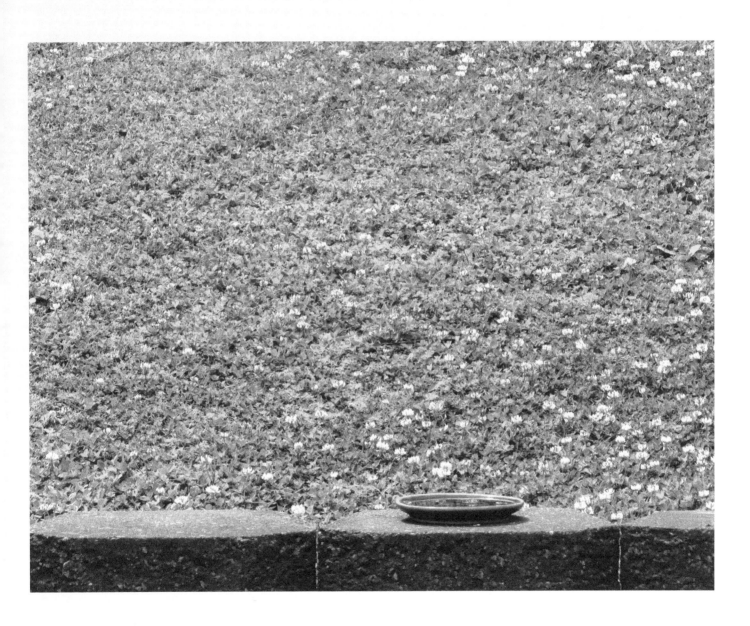

We see and enjoy the radiant soothing colours of nature in all its glorious hues.

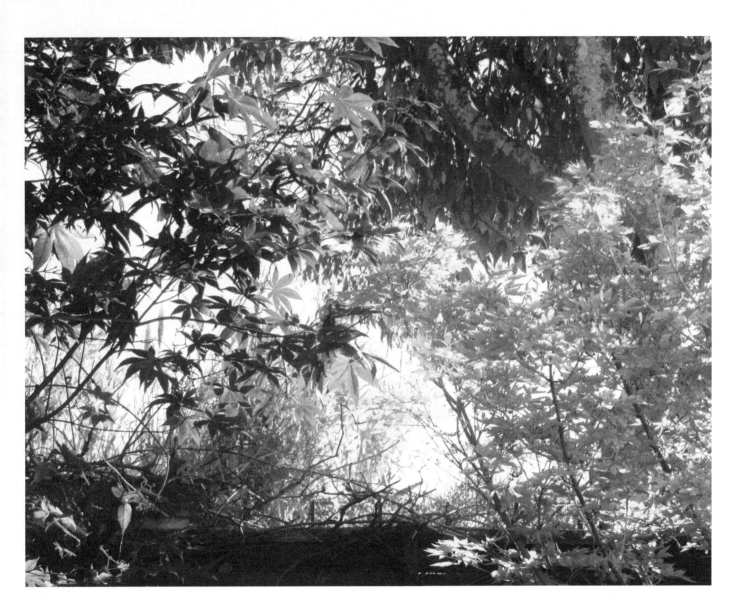

We smell the deliciously calming aroma of our flowers.

We hear the early morning chirping of birds as they welcome each new day, hopping from tree to tree in delight.

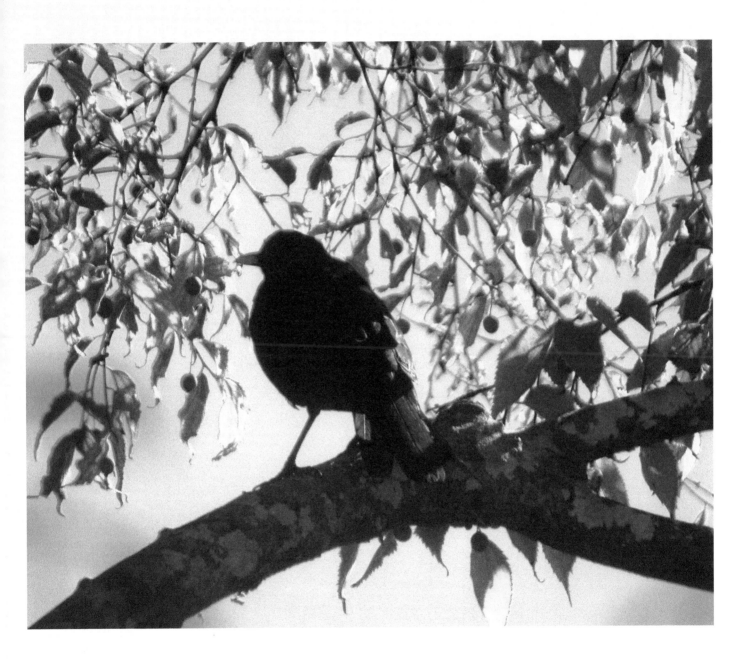

Mindful living is so much fun. Let's mindfully work, laugh and dance today. It will also help us skillfully maneuver through emotions and situations, specially during those difficult moments.

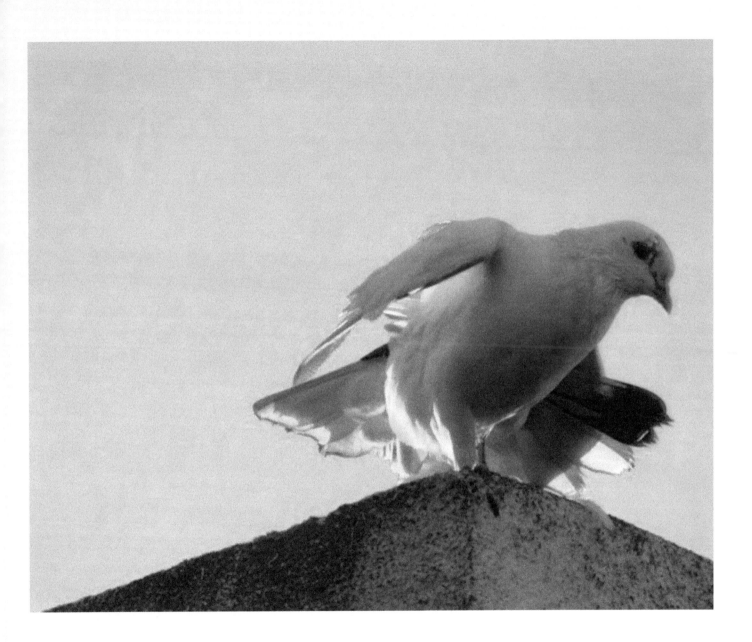

However, our pace of life may leave little room for what is essential—our sleep.

Sleep routines can be difficult: Long school days, overloaded work days, stressful experiences, maintaining and nurturing relationships. But sleep organises our thoughts and our emotions so our mind can be clear to think and the body is at peace.

Let's turn off the light, get comfy in our beds and yes, sleep.

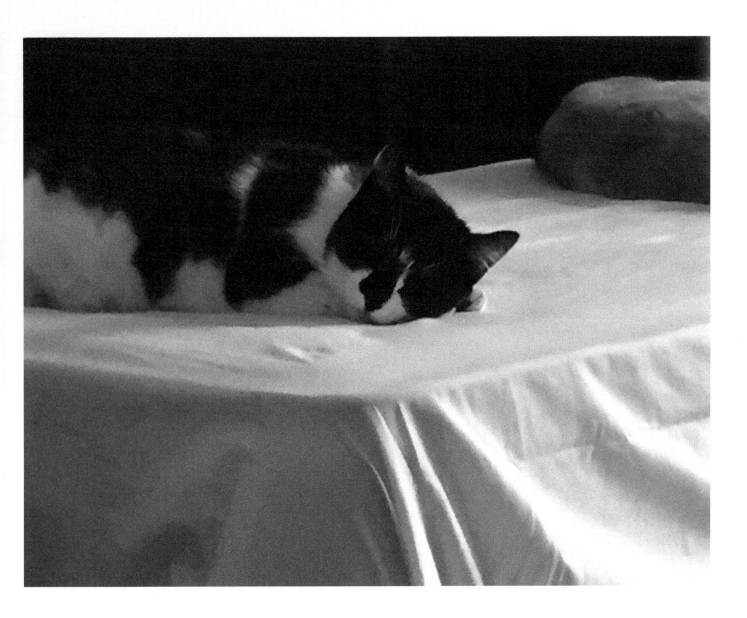

Digital technology has shaped the 21st century. While it facilitates connections with one another, it is love that truly connects us.

To love - whether as a child, parent, friend or person is an incredible emotion. It opens our hearts and gives meaning to life.

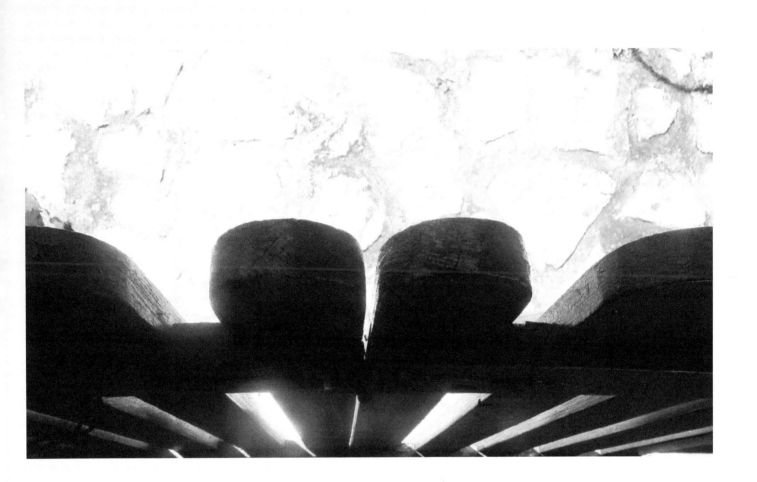

As tasks are preformed and required at a faster pace during our day, mindful leadership and being mindful at our workplace and in our lives has become ever more important.

Reflection is the key that will help us to learn from our mistakes. And to understand that to let our lives be consumed by what we have to do, is to allow the wonders of the world to slip by us.

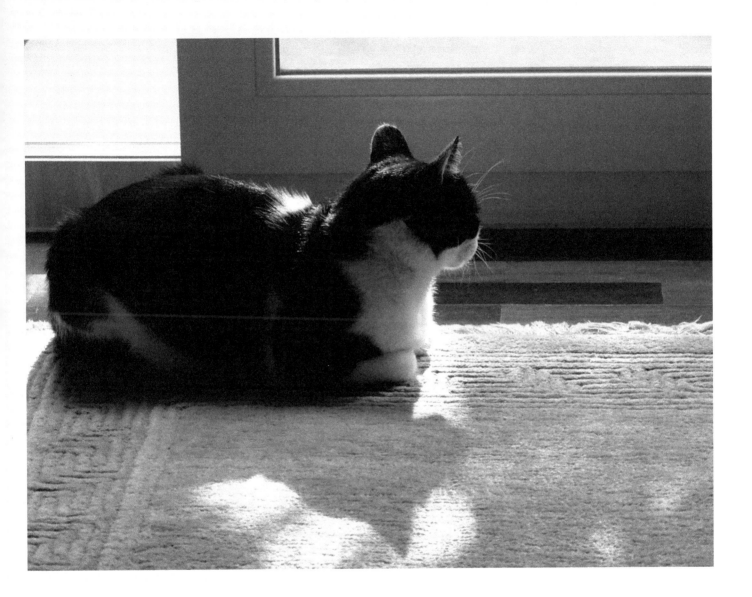

Within our lives, are we able to empathize with love, and move beyond indifference?

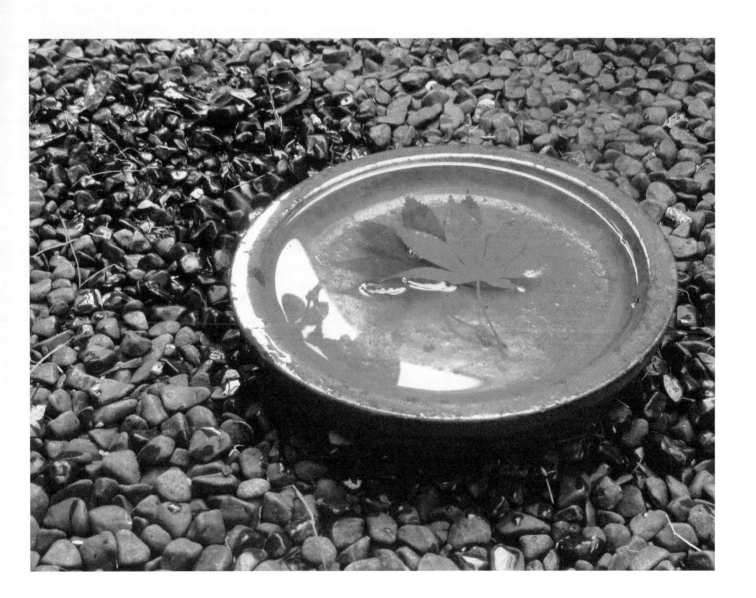

This takes us to another question: In a world with such beauty, why is it difficult to love one another?

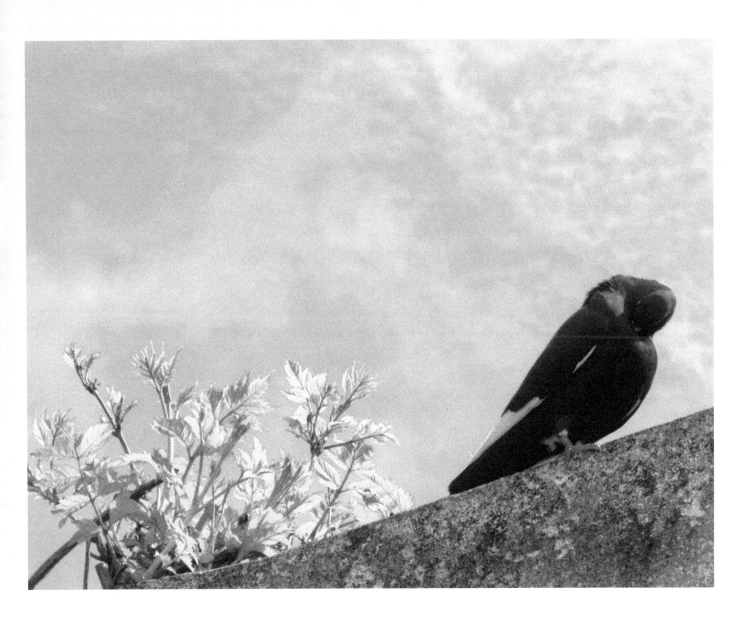

Let's look beyond the surface within the depths of our souls. If we see only on the outside we will miss the beauty that lays within.

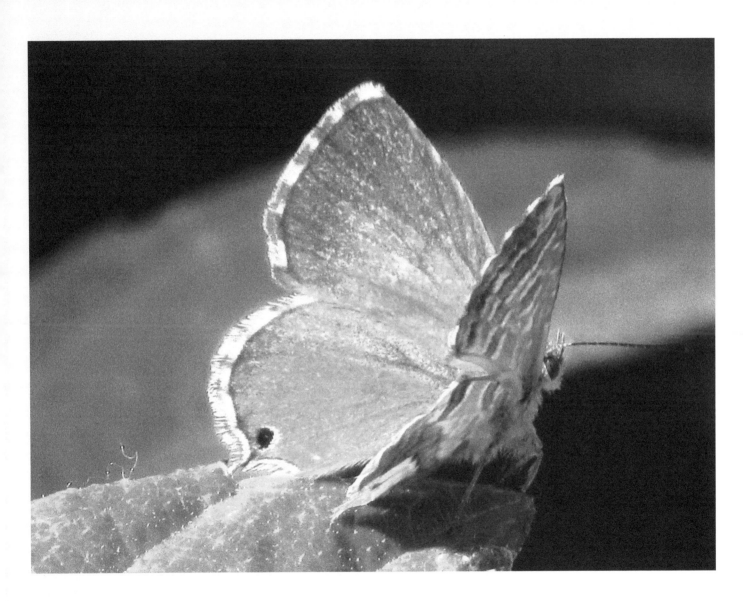

Our beautiful world: inclusive.

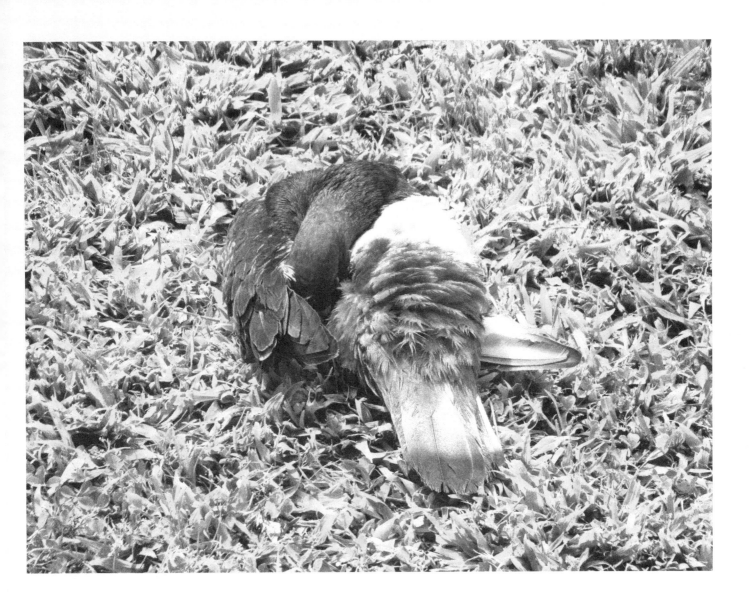

It is an amazing thought that the smallest of crack can allow for incredible growth. We just need to let the light in.

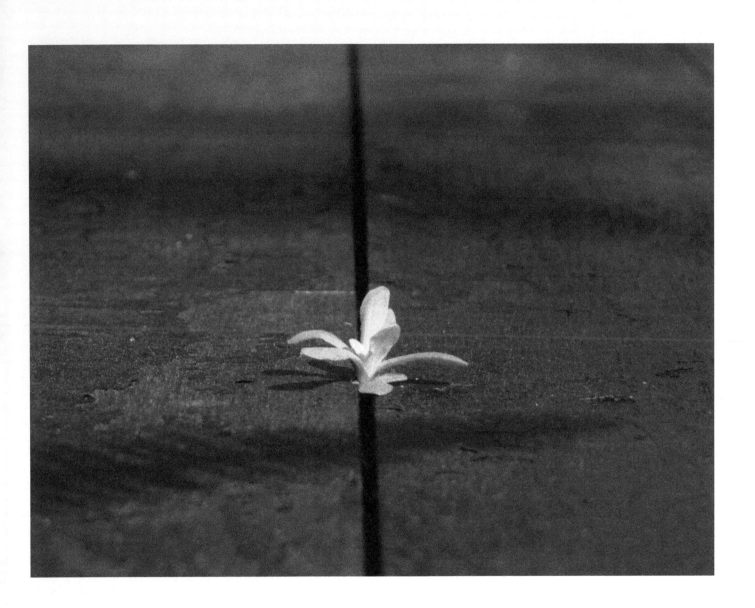

All it takes is love!

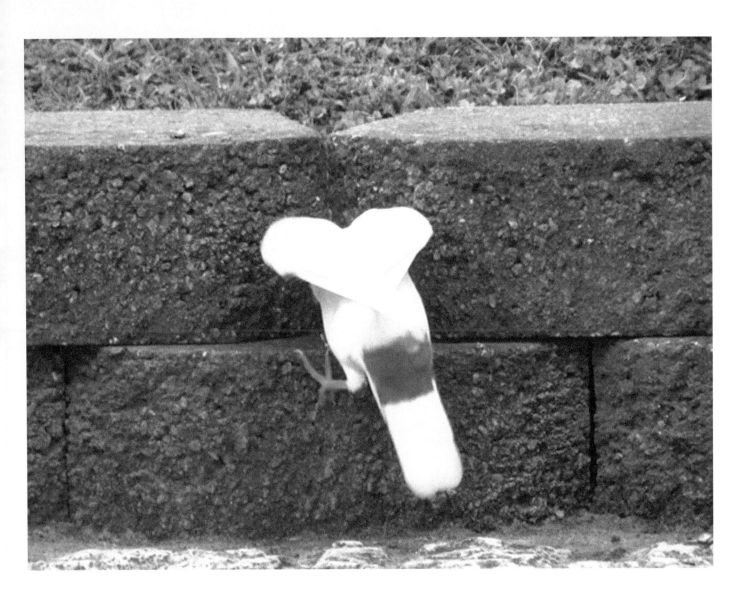

There are times when we may feel challenged by the darkness of our paths. Being mindful helps us see the light as a compass guiding us through our journey, and we have faith.

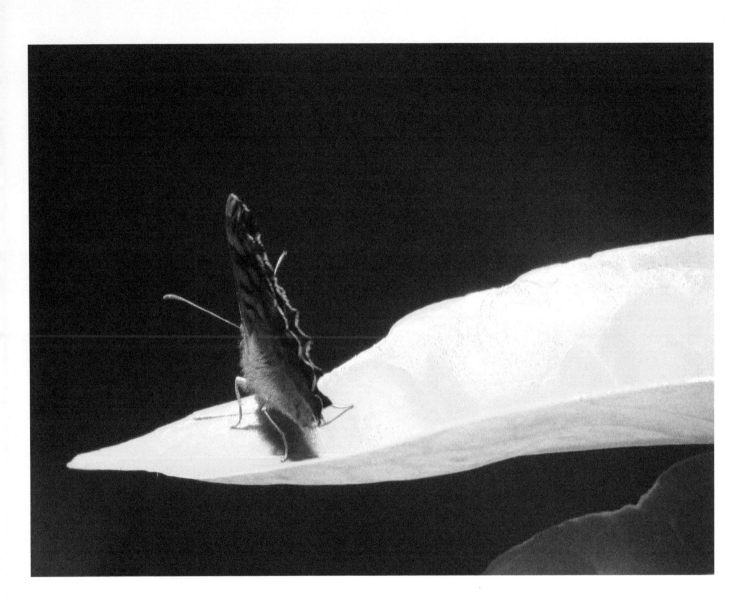

However, the best path isn't necessarily the easiest path.
But we mindfully persevere and have faith.

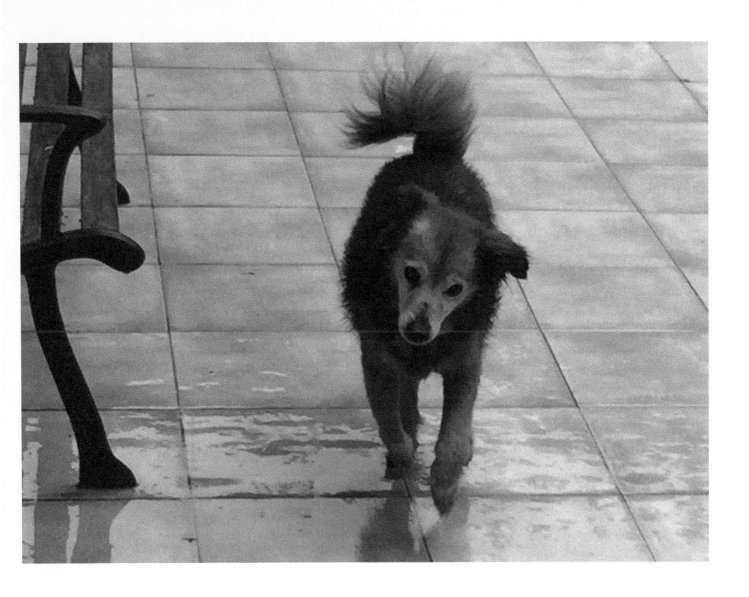

For there is warmth even in the coldest of moments—human kindness is real.

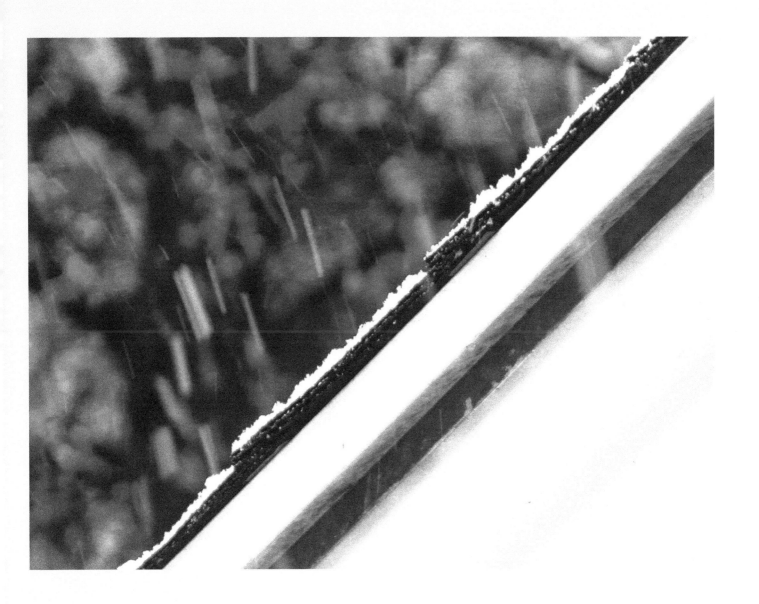

Friendship is a precious gift. It stirs the heart and warms the soul. Let's mindfully share, make the call and extend our hand.

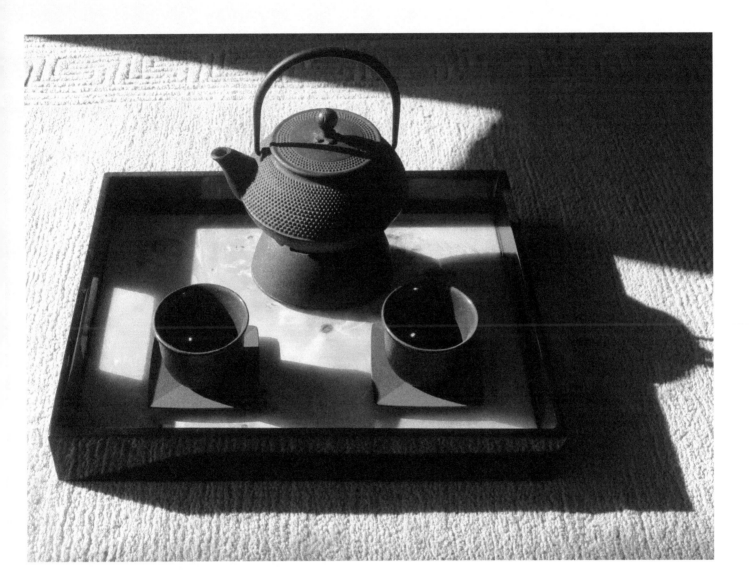

As the colder blanket of winter is replaced by the peaceful colours of spring, one cannot help but feel hopeful as baby robins flutter their wings against the gentle warmer breeze and tufts of green unfold into leaves.

This feeling of rebirth can be translated into our own lives if we mindfully allow ourselves to blossom. Nature is our greatest teacher and also our greatest healer!

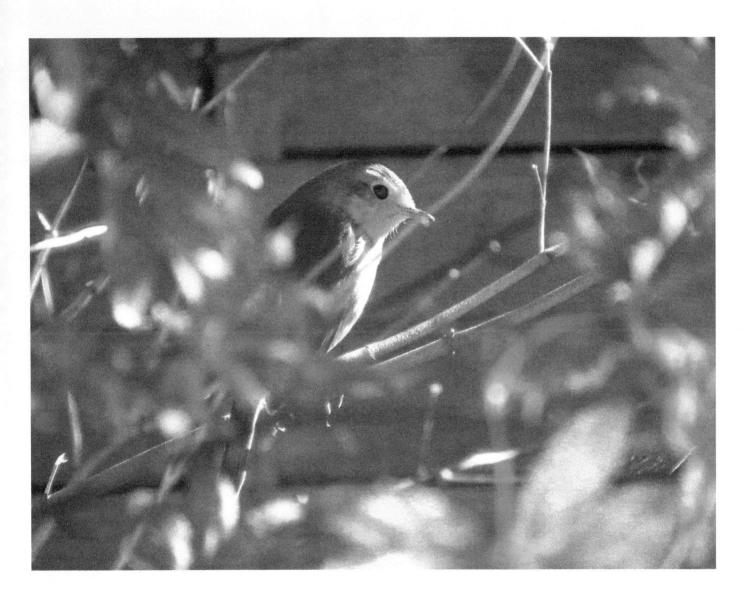

As the light gently nudges the darkness away, we begin to see. We see the wonders of our world, we dream of how wonderful our world can & should be for all and just as importantly - we learn to see ourselves.

However, as we witness more frequent extreme weather conditions, we also need to see our planet. What can we do to slow down global warming and help safe guard our world for generations to come?

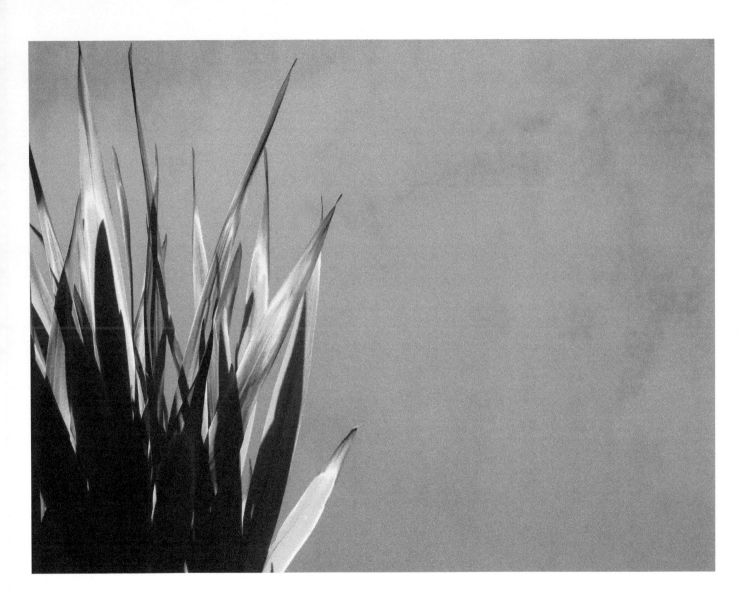

Ocean pollution is a reality. Can you imagine a fish trying to swim home?

Let's be mindful and help save our oceans: choose paper over plastic, recycle, reuse and spread the word. There is no effort too small as we can and need to make the difference.

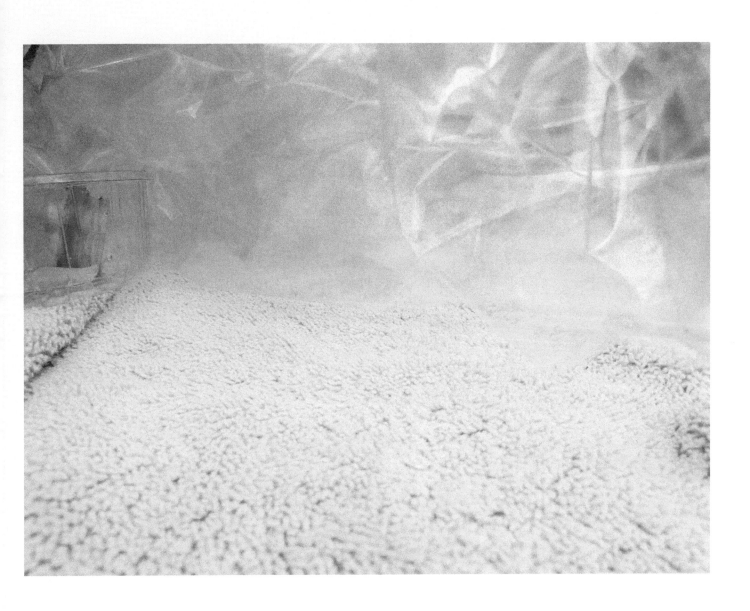

Caring for our plants, our trees and our world is a pleasure but also our responsibility. Together, we can strive to be mindful caretakers of our world.

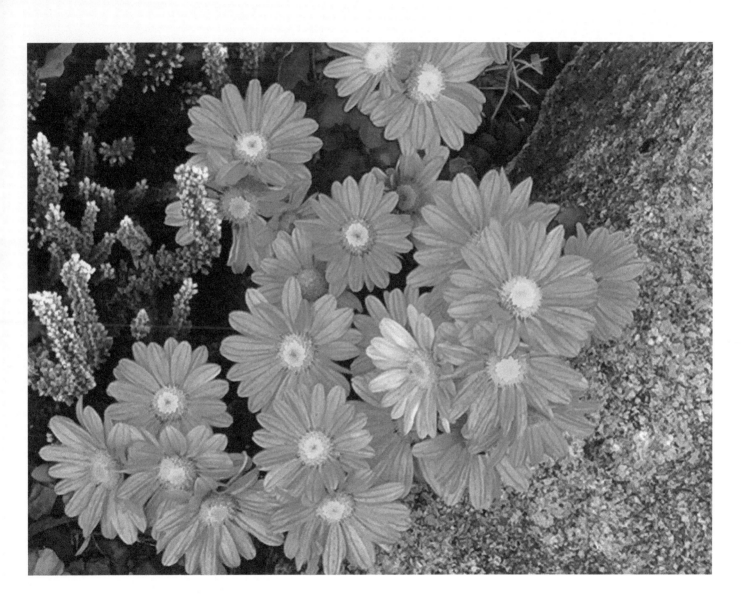

Most of us aspire to live a happy, content and meaningful life, right? It's not that difficult if we remember the most important—the privilege of just being alive.

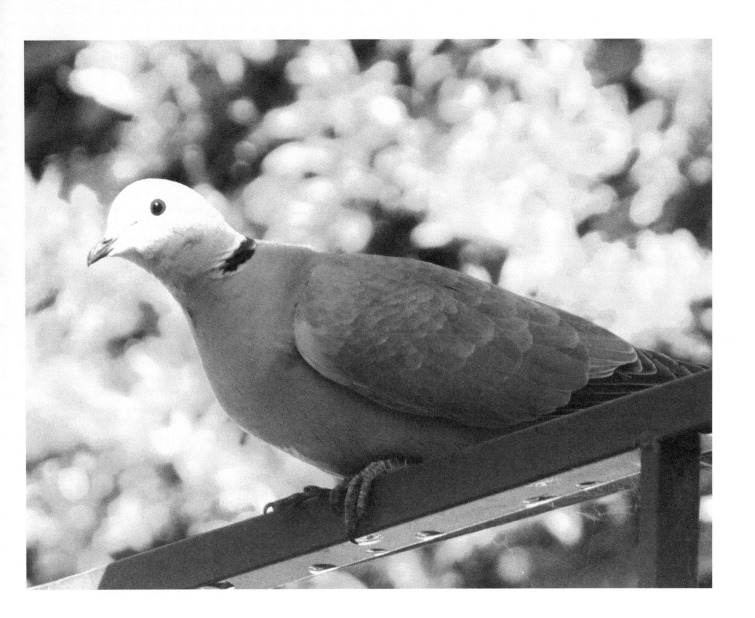

Life spans are increasing at a wonderful pace. Medical advancement is doing its part, but staying healthy also means moving around. Search, experiment and find your activity, not a chore but one that is fun!

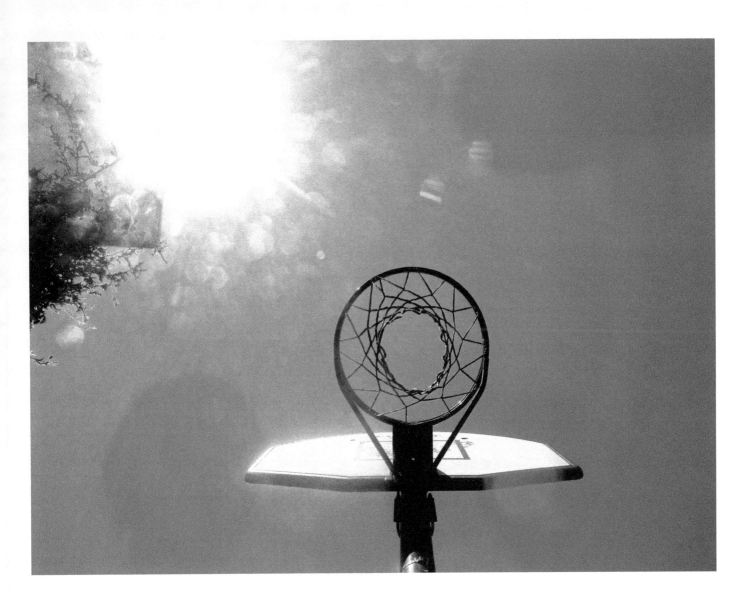

However, what we put into our bodies is essential. Mindful eating helps us make the right choices.

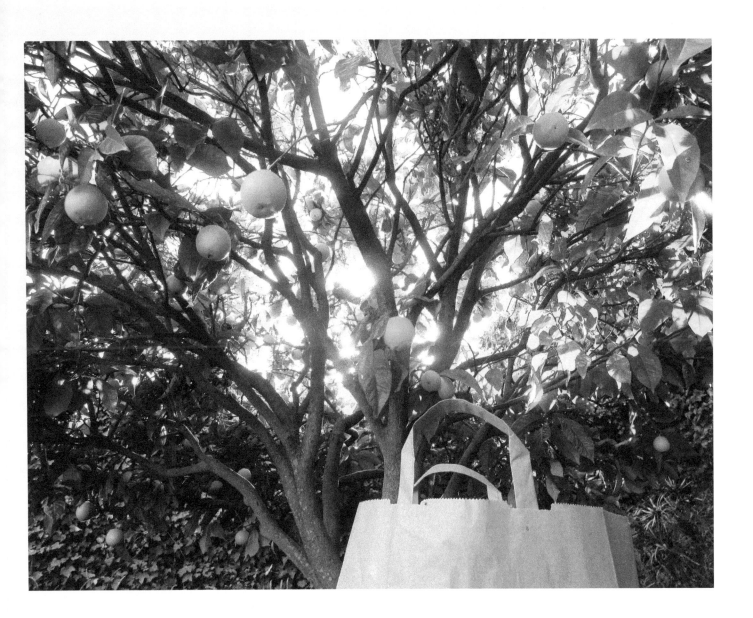

As we take care of our physical wellbeing, what does it take to stay mentally healthy?

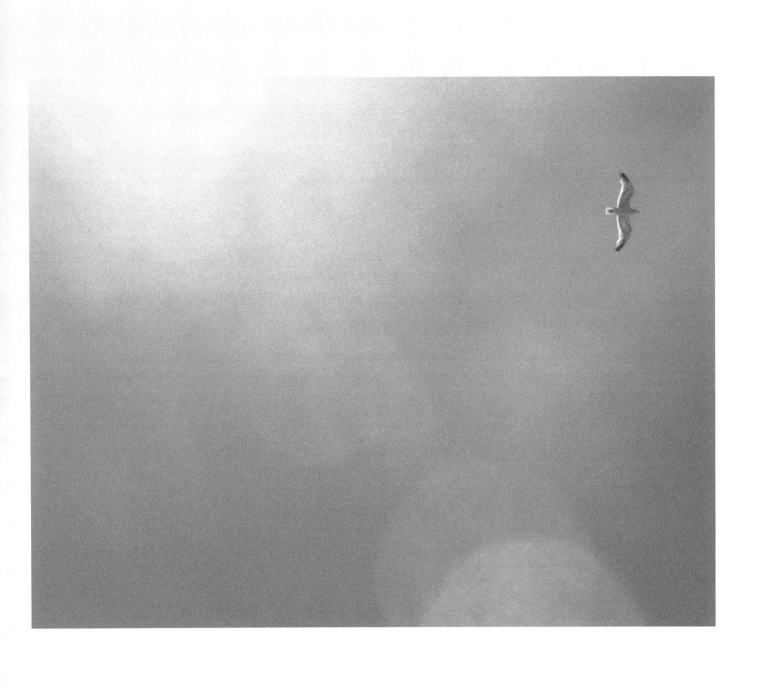

Digital technology is exciting, but it has the potential to create a false illusion that may one day become our reality. Being mindful is essential: Do we reply with kindness, thoughtfulness and respect? Are we conscious of the hours we and our children spend daily on our phones and computers?

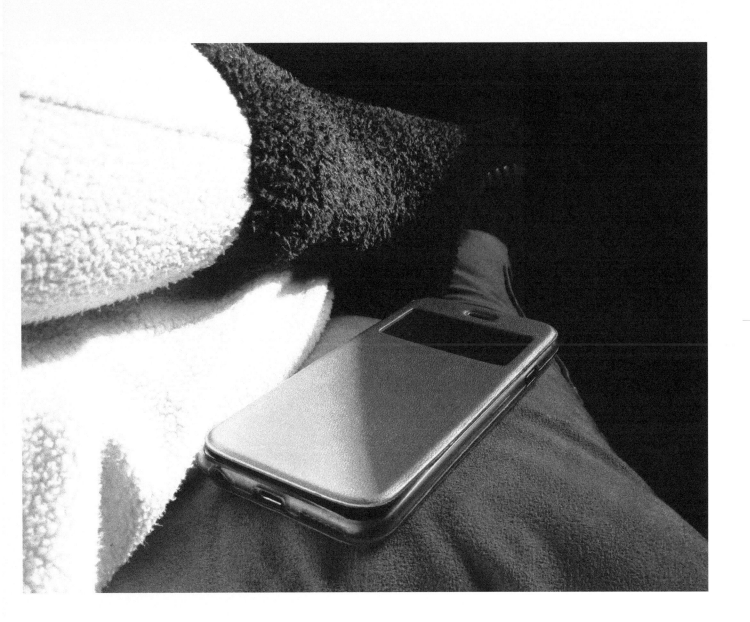

Are we able to unplug, relax and enjoy the silence? True relaxation comes from our ability to hear, see, smell, touch and feel our world.

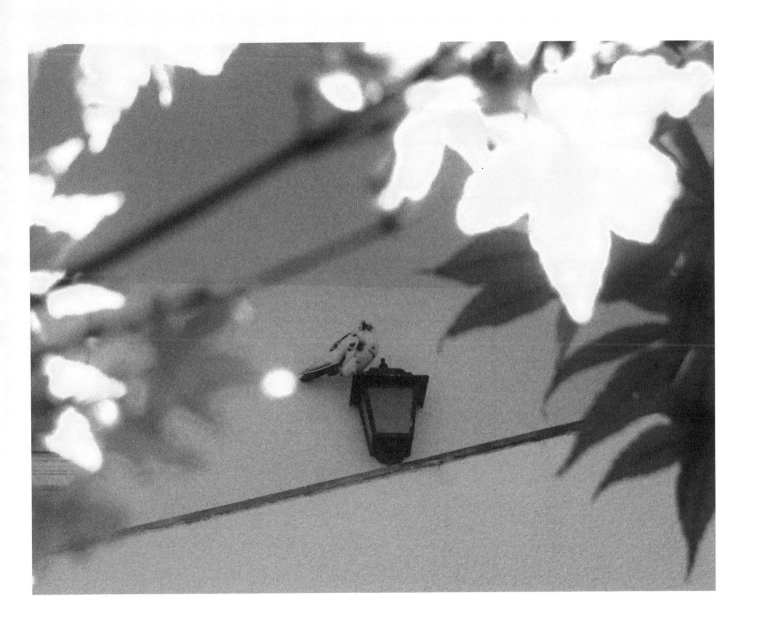

Our world is made up of over 7 billion people, but how many do we trust? Is it possible for us to expand our trust to others within and between our communities?

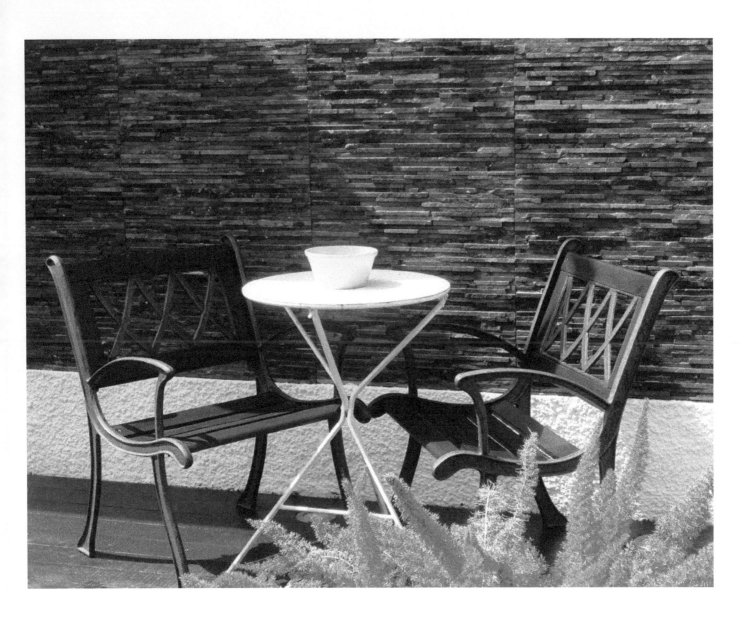

Talking, listening and sharing—Mindful moments help us to connect.

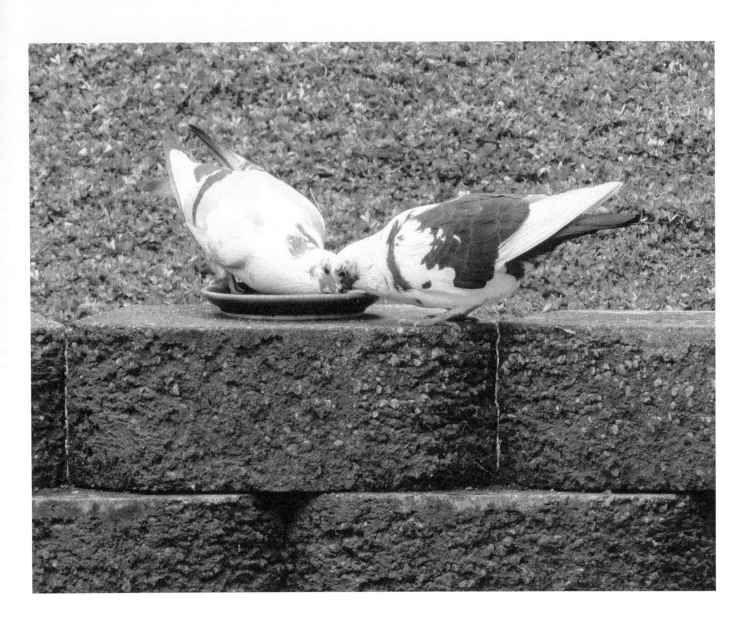

Whether as one species within our chain of evolution or as a human being in our communities—we all share a common denominator: each other.

An amazing thought, isn't it?

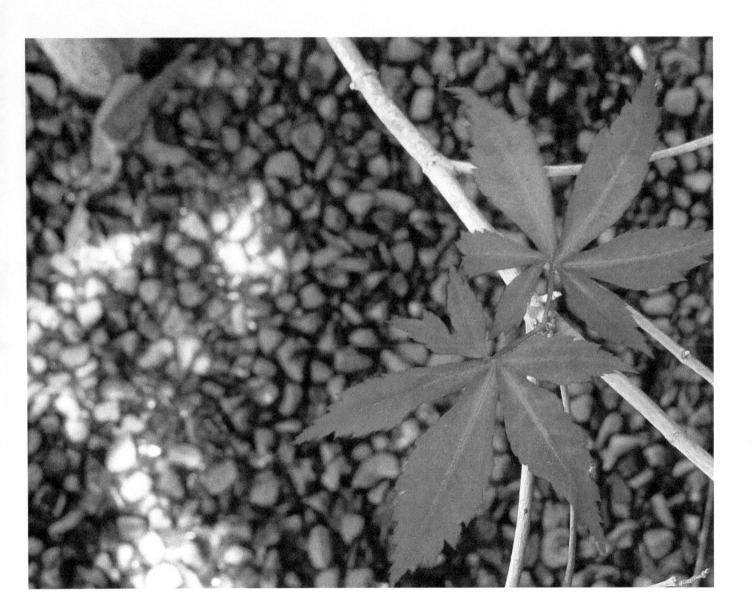

Let's mindfully walk upon our earth hand in hand with kindness and gratefulness, for one cannot exist without the other.

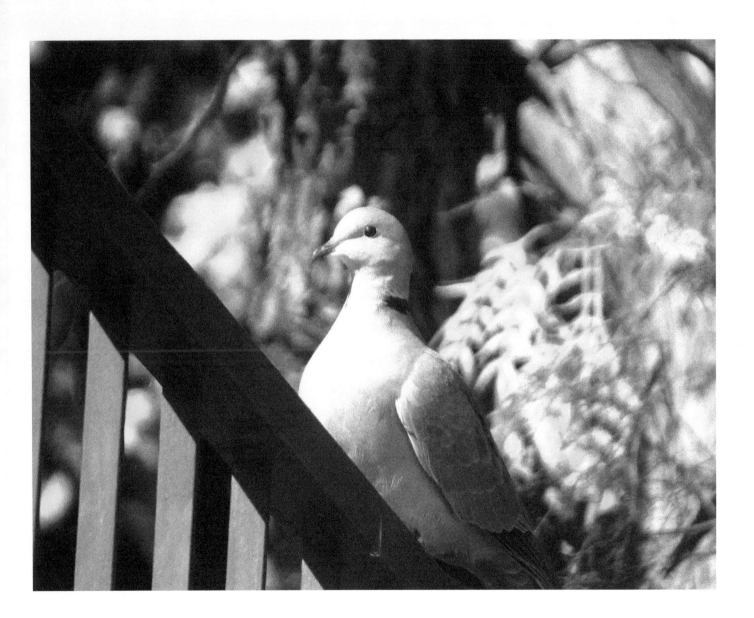

Everything is possible, if we are mindful.

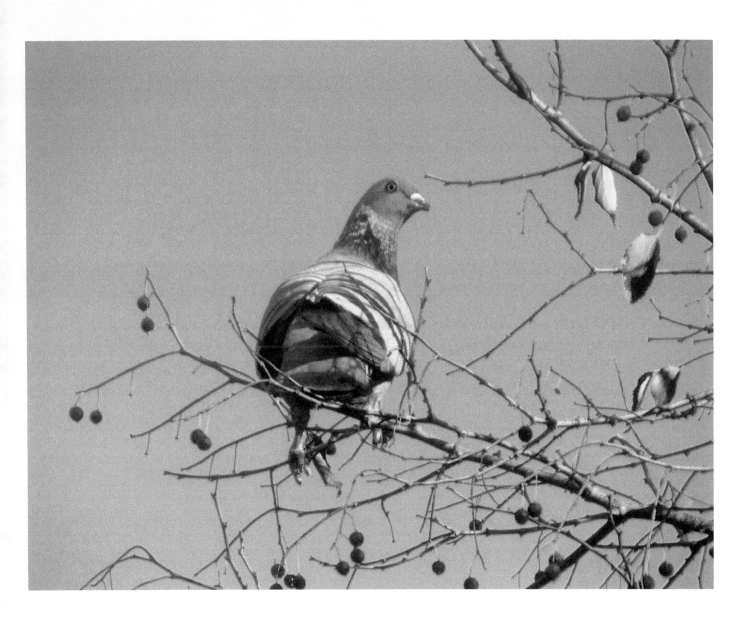

Love and peace are always possible. They are the sources that sustain life in its different forms and shapes. Let us keep love close to our hearts.

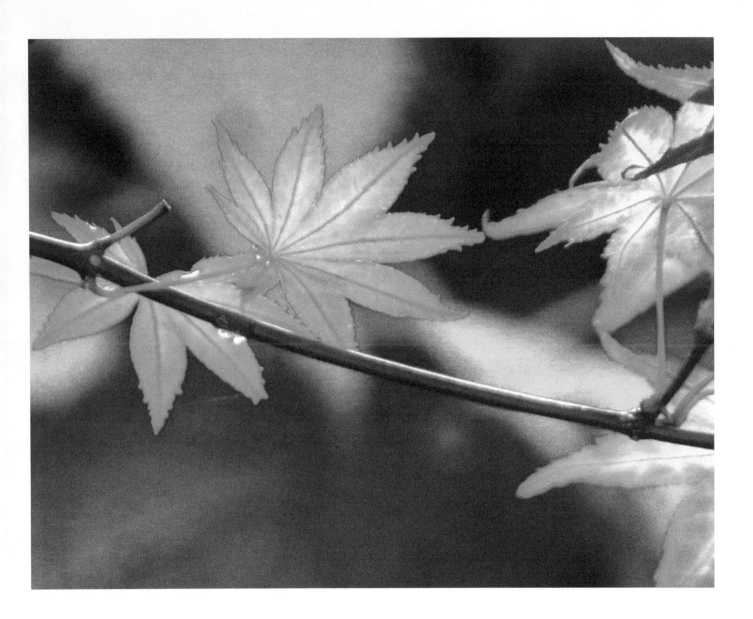

Our world is precious. Let's aspire to *be mindful* and to live our lives with love, respect and care.

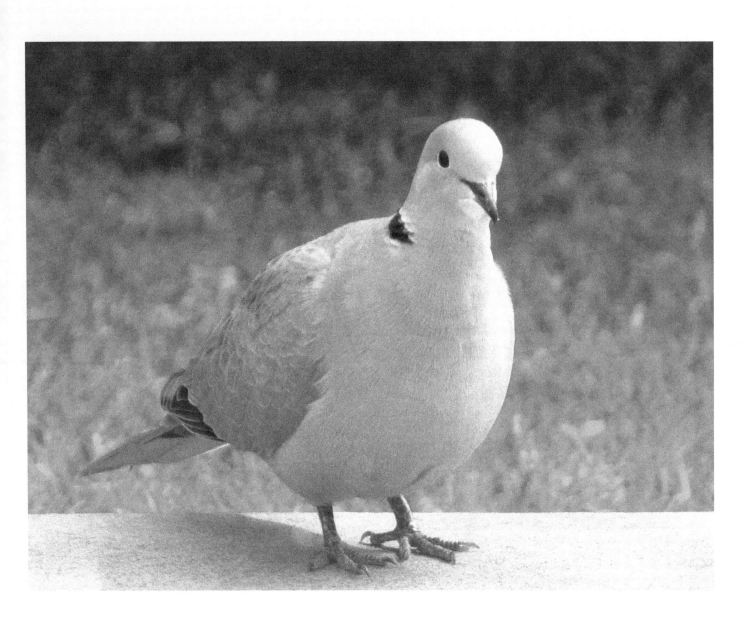

CPSIA information can be obtained
at www.ICGtesting.com
Printed in the USA
BVHW020959110219
539956BV00032B/3622/P

9 781982 217839